The Complete Salad Recipe Cookbook

Table of Contents

The follow Book is reproduced below with the goal of providing information that is as accurate and reliable as possible. Regardless, purchasing this Book can be seen as consent to the fact that both the publisher and the author of this book are in no way experts on the topics discussed within and that any recommendations or suggestions that are made herein are for entertainment purposes only. Professionals should be consulted as needed prior to undertaking any of the action endorsed herein.

This declaration is deemed fair and valid by both the American Bar Association and the Committee of Publishers Association and is legally binding throughout the United States.

Furthermore, the transmission, duplication or reproduction of any of the following work including specific information will be considered an illegal act irrespective of if it is done electronically or in print. This extends to creating a secondary or tertiary copy of the work or a recorded copy and is only allowed with express written consent from the Publisher. All additional right reserved.

The information in the following pages is broadly considered to be a truthful and accurate account of facts and as such any inattention, use or misuse of the information in question by the reader will render any resulting actions solely under their purview. There are no scenarios in which the publisher or the original author of this work can be in any fashion deemed liable for any hardship or damages that may befall them after undertaking information described herein.

Additionally, the information in the following pages is intended only for informational purposes and should thus be thought of as universal. As befitting its nature, it is presented without assurance regarding its prolonged validity or interim quality. Trademarks that are mentioned are done without written consent and can in no way be considered an endorsement from the trademark holder.

BONUS:

As a way of saying thank you for purchasing my book, please use your link below to claim your 3 FREE Cookbooks on Health, Fitness & Dieting Instantly

https://bit.ly/2MkqTit

You can also share your link with your friends and families whom you think that can benefit from the cookbooks or you can forward them the link as a gift!

Chapter 1: Traditional Salad Recipes

Classic three bean salad

Total Prep & Cooking Time: 9 hours
Yields: 6 Servings

What to Use

- ☒ Pepper (as desired)
- ☒ Salt (as desired)
- ☒ Green beans (16 oz. drained)
- ☒ White sugar (.25 c)
- ☒ Vegetable oil (.5 c)
- ☒ Vinegar (.5 c)
- ☒ Pimento peppers (4 oz. drained, chopped)
- ☒ Green bell pepper (1 c chopped)
- ☒ Celery (1 c chopped)
- ☒ Onion (1 c chopped)
- ☒ Red kidney beans (16 oz. drained)
- ☒ Yellow wax beans (16 oz. drained)
- ☒ Green beans (16 oz. drained)

What to Do

- ☒ In a serving bowl, combine the green bell pepper, celery, onion, kidney beans, yellow wax beans, pimento peppers and green beans and mix well to combine thoroughly.
- ☒ In a saucepan, combine the pepper, salt, sugar oil and vinegar and mix well before placing the saucepan on the stove over a burner turned to a high heat and allow it boil, stirring throughout so the sugar dissolves.
- ☒ Toss salad with dressing to coat before placing the serving dish in the refrigerator for at least 8 hours to allow flavors to properly mix.

Classic Israeli cucumber and tomato salad

Total Prep & Cooking Time: 20 minutes
Yields: 6 Servings

What to Use

- Pepper (as desired)
- Salt (as desired)
- Lemon juice (2 T)
- Olive oil (.5 c)
- Garlic (2 T chopped)
- Red bell pepper (1 diced, seeded)
- Purple onion (.5 diced)
- Roma tomatoes (4 diced, seeded)
- English cucumbers (4 diced)

What to Do

- Combine the pepper, salt, lemon juice and olive oil together in a small bowl and mix well to combine thoroughly.
- Add the English cucumbers, Roma tomatoes, purple onion, red bell pepper and chopped garlic to a serving bowl and mix well.
- Toss with dressing to ensure it is fully coated.

Classic seven-layer salad

Total Prep & Cooking Time: 50 minutes
Yields: 8 Servings

What to Use

- Pepper (as desired)
- Salt (as desired)
- Bacon (.5 c cooked, crumbled)
- Water chestnuts (4 oz. drained, sliced)
- Peas (10 oz. frozen, thawed)
- Black olives (6 oz. drained, sliced)
- Roma tomatoes (to taste, chopped)
- Iceberg lettuce (4 c torn)
- Mayonnaise (1.25 c)
- Cheddar cheese (2 c shredded)

What to Do

- In a small bowl, combine the mayonnaise and cheddar cheese and combine thoroughly.
- In a glass serving bowl, form the lettuce into a firm layer on the bottom of the bowl. Top that layer with a layer of tomatoes, followed by a layer of black olive, then a layer of peas and then finally a layer of water chestnuts. Top with a layer of cheddar cheese and then finish it off with a layer of bacon.
- Top the bacon layer with a firm layer of plastic wrap and then place the salad in the refrigerator for at least 30 minutes.
- Serve chilled.

Classic cucumber salad

Total Prep & Cooking Time: 135 minutes
Yields: 6 Servings

What to Use

- ☒ Pepper (as desired)
- ☒ Salt (as desired)
- ☒ White onion (1 sliced into rings)
- ☒ Tomatoes (3 wedged)
- ☒ Cucumbers (3 sliced, peeled)
- ☒ Sugar (.25 c)
- ☒ Vegetable oil (.25 c)
- ☒ White vinegar (.5 c distilled)
- ☒ Water (1 c)

What to Do

- ☒ In a large serving bowl, whisk together the pepper, salt, sugar, oil, vinegar and water before adding in the onion, tomatoes and cucumber and tossing to coat.
- ☒ Cover the serving bowl with plastic wrap and let it chill in the refrigerator for at least two hours prior to serving.

Classic German potato salad

Total Prep & Cooking Time: 4 hours
Yields: 10 Servings

What to Use

- ☒ Pepper (as desired)
- ☒ Salt (as desired)
- ☒ Sugar (2 T)

- ☒ Water (.5 c)
- ☒ White vinegar (1 c)
- ☒ Garlic (4 cloves minced)
- ☒ Sweet onions (2 diced)
- ☒ Bacon (1 lb.)
- ☒ Red potatoes (5 lbs. diced)

What to Do

- ☒ Add the potatoes to a pot before filling the pot with water so the potatoes are completely covered. Season as desired before placing the pot on the stove over a burner turned to a high heat. Allow the water to boil before reducing the heat to low/medium and letting the potatoes simmer for about 20 minutes or until they are nice and tender. Drain the potatoes before adding them to a slow cooker.
- ☒ Add the bacon to a skillet before placing the skillet on the stove over a burner turned to a high/medium heat and letting it cook about 10 minutes. Crumble the bacon and add it to the potatoes.
- ☒ Reheat the skillet to a medium heat, while retaining the bacon grease. Add in the onions and let them cook 5 minutes before adding in the garlic and cooking 2 more minutes. Add the results to the slow cooker.
- ☒ In a small bowl, mix together the salt, sugar, water and vinegar and combine thoroughly before adding it to the top of the slow cooker and mixing well.
- ☒ Allow the slow cooker to cook, covered, for 4 hours on a low heat.

Classic Greek salad

Total Prep & Cooking Time: 10 minutes
Yields: 8 Servings

What to Use

- ☒ Pepper (as desired)
- ☒ Salt (as desired)
- ☒ Red onion (.5 sliced)
- ☒ Sun-dried tomatoes (.3 c drained, oil reserved)
- ☒ Roma tomatoes (3 c diced)
- ☒ Black olives (1 c pitted, sliced)
- ☒ Feta cheese (1.5 c crumbled)
- ☒ Cucumbers (3 sliced, seeded)

What to Do

- ☒ Combine all of the ingredients in a serving bowl and mix well.
- ☒ Toss with dressing as desired.
- ☒ Cover the serving bowl with plastic wrap and chill prior to serving.

Classic Mediterranean salad

Total Prep & Cooking Time: 50 minutes
Yields: 4 Servings

What to Use

- ☒ Pepper (as desired)
- ☒ Salt (as desired)
- ☒ Lemon (1 zested)
- ☒ Oregano (2 tsp. dried)

- ☒ Garlic (2 cloves minced)
- ☒ White vinegar (1 T)
- ☒ Parsley (2 T)
- ☒ Extra-virgin olive oil (.25 c)
- ☒ Lemons (2 juiced)
- ☒ Zucchini (3 spiralized)
- ☒ Kalamata olive (.5 c pitted, halved)
- ☒ Cherry tomatoes (1 c halved)
- ☒ Artichoke hearts (10 oz. chopped, drained)

What to Do

- ☒ Combine the zucchini, olives, tomatoes and artichoke hearts in a serving bowl and mix well.
- ☒ In a separate bowl, combine the pepper, salt, lemon zest, oregano, garlic, vinegar, parsley, olive oil and lemon juice and mix well to combine thoroughly.
- ☒ Add the dressing to the salad and toss to coat.
- ☒ Top the zucchini with feta cheese prior to serving.

Chapter 2: Quick and Easy Salad Recipes

Chef Salad

Total Prep & Cooking Time: 15 minutes
Yields: 4 Servings

What to Use

- ☒ Pepper (as desired)
- ☒ Salt (as desired)
- ☒ Monterey Jack cheese (4 oz. shredded)
- ☒ Radishes (6 sliced thin)
- ☒ Avocado (1 pitted, sliced)
- ☒ Boston lettuce (1 head large)
- ☒ Honey (1 T)
- ☒ Sour cream (.3 c)
- ☒ Carrots (4 sliced)
- ☒ Alfalfa sprouts (1 c)
- ☒ Roasted turkey (1 lb. sliced, torn)
- ☒ Apple cider vinegar (2 T)
- ☒ Buttermilk (.3 c low-fat)

What to Do

- ☒ Combine the cheese, carrots, radishes, sprouts, avocado, turkey and lettuce in a serving bowl and mix well.
- ☒ In a small separate bowl combine the pepper, salt, honey, vinegar, sour cream and buttermilk and whisk well.
- ☒ Toss with dressing as desired prior to serving.

Thai Salad

Total Prep & Cooking Time: 20 minutes
Yields: 4 Servings

What to Use

- ☒ Pepper (as desired)
- ☒ Salt (as desired)
- ☒ English cucumber (1 halved, peeled, chopped)
- ☒ Serrano chili (chopped)
- ☒ Lime juice (.25 c)
- ☒ Safflower oil (2 T)
- ☒ Mint leaves (1 handful chopped)
- ☒ Brown sugar (2 tsp.)
- ☒ Fish sauce (2 T)
- ☒ Red onion (.5 sliced thin)
- ☒ Napa cabbage (1 head)
- ☒ Pork chops (4)

What to Do

- ☒ Place a skillet over a burner turned to a high heat and let it heat up for 5 minutes before adding half of the cabbage and letting it cook about 3 minutes, flipping in the middle.
- ☒ Remove the cabbage from the skillet, add 1 T oil and then add in the pork and cook each side about 2 minutes until its internal temperature is at least 140 degrees F.
- ☒ Remove the pork from the skillet and slice it once it has cooled slightly and combine all of the ingredients in a serving dish and toss to combine before dividing evenly among the plates with the cabbage on the bottom.

Chicken salad with green beans and cherries

Total Prep & Cooking Time: 15 minutes
Yields: 4 Servings

What to Use

- ☒ Pepper (as desired)
- ☒ Salt (as desired)
- ☒ Cherries (.3 c dried)
- ☒ Arugula (5 oz.)
- ☒ Apricot jam (1 T)
- ☒ Green beans (.5 lb. trimmed)
- ☒ Chicken breast cutlets (1 lb.)
- ☒ Almonds (.25 c sliced)
- ☒ Radicchio (1 head, shredded, cored)
- ☒ Dijon mustard (1 T)
- ☒ Red wine vinegar (3 T)
- ☒ Olive oil (3T)

What to Do

- ☒ Add 1 T oil to a skillet before placing it on a burner turned to a high heat before adding in the seasoned chicken and cooking it about 1.5 minutes per side until it reaches an internal temperature of 165 degrees F. Remove the chicken from the skillet and slice it when cool.
- ☒ Add 2 inches slated water to a saucepan and place it on a burner turned to a high heat and allow it to boil before adding in the green beans and letting them cook about 4 minutes. Rinse under cold water and drain.
- ☒ In a small bowl, combine 2 T oil, mustard, jam and vinegar and whisk well before seasoning as desired
- ☒ Add the remaining ingredients to a serving bowl and toss well.

☒ Plate the salad, top with the chicken and then the dressing prior to serving.

Steak salad

Total Prep & Cooking Time: 20 minutes
Yields: 4 Servings

What to Use

☒ Pepper (as desired)
☒ Salt (as desired)
☒ Carrots (3 sliced)
☒ Red leaf lettuce (1 head torn)
☒ Dijon mustard (1 T)
☒ Olive oil (2 T)
☒ Radishes (8 quartered)
☒ Garlic (1 clove minced)
☒ White wine vinegar (2 T)
☒ Snap peas (8 oz. halved, steamed)
☒ Skirt steak (1 lb. halved)

What to Do

☒ Heat your broiler before placing the steak on top of a baking sheet lined with tinfoil (seasoned as desired) and broiling the steak for 4 minutes. Remove the steak from the broil and tent it in the tinfoil to keep it warm.
☒ Combine the garlic, mustard, vinegar and oil and whisk well to combine thoroughly. Toss the lettuce using half the dressing.
☒ Slice the steak and place it and the remaining ingredients on top of the tossed salad. Top with dressing prior to serving.

Chicken salad with pistachios and feta

Total Prep & Cooking Time: 20 minutes
Yields: 4 Servings

What to Use

- ☒ Pepper (as desired)
- ☒ Salt (as desired)
- ☒ Feta (4 oz. crumbled)
- ☒ Parsley (.5 c)
- ☒ Coriander (1 tsp.)
- ☒ Olive oil (.25 c + 1 T)
- ☒ Navel oranges (2 halved, sliced thin)
- ☒ Scallions (1 bunch sliced thin)
- ☒ Romaine lettuce (1 head chopped)
- ☒ Chicken cutlets (1 lb.)
- ☒ White wine vinegar (.25 c)
- ☒ Pistachios (.5 c)

What to Do

- ☒ Add the pistachios to a skillet before placing the skillet on a burner turned to a medium heat. All them to cook for 7 minutes, regularly stirring.
- ☒ Once they have cooled place them in a bowl and whisk in vinegar, .25 c oil, salt and pepper and mix well.
- ☒ Add the rest of the of the oil to the skillet before seasoning the chicken and cooking it about 2 minutes per side or until its internal temperature reaches 165 degrees F. Slice the chicken once it has cooled.
- ☒ Combine the scallions, parsley, lettuce and pistachios with the dressing and toss well. Plate the salad before topping with oranges, feta and chicken.

Spinach salad with salmon

Total Prep & Cooking Time: 15 minutes
Yields: 4 Servings

What to Use

- Pepper (as desired)
- Salt (as desired)
- Pecans (.25 c)
- Grape tomatoes (1 pint halved)
- Balsamic vinaigrette (.25 c)
- Goat cheese (.75 c crumbled)
- Baby spinach (10 oz.)
- Salmon fillet (4 skin removed)

What to Do

- ☒ Place the salmon on a lined baking sheet and season as desired before broiling the fish about 7 minutes. Flake the fish once it has cooled.
- ☒ Combine the remaining ingredients together and plate before topping with the fish, pecans and goat cheese. Drizzle with vinaigrette prior to serving.

Zucchini salad with chicken

Total Prep & Cooking Time: 30 minutes
Yields: 4 Servings

What to Use

- Pepper (as desired)
- Salt (as desired)
- Mint (.25 c chopped)

- Pecans (.75 c chopped)
- Spinach (8 oz. chopped)
- Zucchini (1.25 lbs. sliced thin)
- Lemon juice (.25 c)
- Parmesan cheese (.25 c grated)
- Red onion (.5 sliced thin)
- Chicken breast (1 lb.)
- Olive oil (.25 c + 1 T)

What to Do

☒ Combine the lemon juice and .25 c oil in a serving bowl and mix well before adding in the zucchini and tossing to coat. Allow it to remain in the mixture while the chicken cooks.

☒ Add the rest of the oil to a skillet before placing the skillet on a burner set to a medium heat. Season the chicken as desired before adding it to the skillet and letting it cook until it reaches an internal temperature of 165 degrees.

☒ Add all of the ingredients to the serving bowl and toss well prior to serving.

Chapter 3: Group Salad Recipes

Zucchini salad with Arugula

Total Prep & Cooking Time: 20 minutes
Yields: 10 Servings

What to Use

- Pepper (as desired)
- Salt (as desired)
- Basil leaves (25)
- Arugula (5 oz.)
- Balsamic vinaigrette (.25 c + 1 T)
- Grape tomatoes (10 oz.)
- Mozzarella cheese (2.5 lbs. cubed)
- Zucchini (5 spiralized)

What to Do

- Add the vinaigrette, tomatoes, mozzarella and zucchini in a serving bowl and mix well. Place in the refrigerator until you are ready to serve.
- Prior to serving mix in the basil and arugula.

Caesar salad sandwich

Total Prep & Cooking Time: 25 minutes
Yields: 10 Servings

What to Use

- Pepper (as desired)
- Salt (as desired)
- Parmesan cheese (1.25 c shredded)

- Caesar salad dressing (2.5 c)
- Romaine lettuce (2.5 heads quartered)
- Tomatoes (2.5 halved)
- Garlic (5 cloves halved)
- Olive oil (.5 c + 2 T)
- Baguettes (2.5)

What to Do

- ☒ Prepare your grill to a low temperature and ensure the grate is oiled.
- ☒ Slice baguettes in quarters and brush using olive oil.
- ☒ Grill the baguette pieces for about 2 minutes per side. Rub the bread with tomatoes and garlic and set it aside.
- ☒ Use the rest of the olive oil to brush the romaine lettuce and then grill it for about 2 minutes per side. Season with salt and set it aside.
- ☒ Place the lettuce on top of the baguette and top with Caesar dressing and Parmesan cheese.

Kale Salad

Total Prep & Cooking Time: 10 minutes
Yields: 10 Servings

What to Use

- Pepper (as desired)
- Salt (as desired)
- Cranberries (1.25 c dried)
- Sunflower seeds (1.25 c)
- Tomato (2.5 diced)
- Kale (2.5 bunches chopped)
- White sugar (2.5 tsp.)

- Olive oil (2 T + 1.5 tsp.)
- Canola oil (2 T + 1.5 tsp.)
- Lemon juice (1.25 c)

What to Do

- ☒ In a serving bowl, whisk together the oil, salt, pepper and lemon juice and combine thoroughly.
- ☒ Mix in the cranberries, sunflower seeds, tomato and kale and toss to combine prior to serving.

Watermelon salad with spinach

Total Prep & Cooking Time: 20 minutes
Yields: 10 Servings

What to Use

- Pepper (as desired)
- Salt (as desired)
- Watermelon chunks (5 c)
- Feta cheese (1.25 c)
- Grape tomatoes (2.5 c halved)
- Red onion (2.5 c sliced thin)
- Baby spinach leaves (5 c)
- Arugula (5 c)
- Balsamic vinegar (1T + 2 tsp.)
- Extra virgin olive oil (.3 c + 2 T)

What to Do

- ☒ In a serving bowl, whisk together the oil, salt, pepper and balsamic vinegar and combine thoroughly.
- ☒ Mix in the tomatoes, onions, spinach and arugula and toss to combine prior to serving. Top with feta cheese and watermelon and serve.

Green Salad

Total Prep & Cooking Time: 10 minutes
Yields: 10 Servings

What to Use

- Pepper (as desired)
- Salt (as desired)
- Feta cheese (5 oz. crumbled)
- Almonds (1.25 c sliced)
- Mixed salad greens (10 c)
- Avocados (2.5 cubed, pitted, peeled)
- Garlic (5 cloves chopped)
- Lemon juice (2.5 tsp.)
- Parsley (2.5 tsp. chopped)
- White sugar (2 pinches)
- Dijon mustard (2 T + 1.5 tsp.)
- White wine vinegar (.25 c + 1 T)
- Olive oil (.5 c + 2 T)

What to Do

- ☒ In a serving bowl, whisk together the oil, vinegar, garlic, lemon juice, parsley, sugar, pepper, salt and mustard and combine thoroughly.
- ☒ Mix in the salad greens and toss to combine prior to serving. Top with feta cheese and sliced almonds and serve.

Salad with cranberry vinaigrette

Total Prep & Cooking Time: 20 minutes
Yields: 10 Servings

What to Use

- Pepper (as desired)
- Salt (as desired)
- Mixed greens (1.25 lbs.)
- Blue cheese (5 oz. crumbled)
- Red onion (.5 sliced thin)
- Water (2 T + 1.5 tsp.)
- Garlic (.5 tsp. minced)
- Dijon mustard (1 T + .75 tsp.)
- Cranberries (.25 c + 1 T)
- Olive oil (.3 c + 1 T + 1 tsp.)
- Red wine vinegar (3 T + 2.25 tsp.)
- Almonds (1.25 c sliced)

What to Do

- ☒ Ensure your oven is heated to 375 degrees F.
- ☒ Place the almonds on a baking sheet in a single layer and place the baking sheet in the oven for 5 minutes.
- ☒ Add the water, pepper, salt, garlic, mustard, cranberries, oil and vinegar to a food processor and process well.
- ☒ Add the blue cheese, onion, almonds and salad greens into a serving bowl, top with the dressing and toss well prior to serving.

Italian salad

Total Prep & Cooking Time: 15 minutes
Yields: 10 Servings

What to Use

- Pepper (as desired)
- Salt (as desired)
- Lemon juice (3 T + 1 tsp.)
- Balsamic vinegar (.3 c + 1 T + 1 tsp.)
- Basil (3 T + 1 tsp.)
- Grapeseed oil (.3 c + 1 T + 1 tsp.)
- Cherry tomatoes (20)
- Green bell pepper (1 sliced)
- Red bell pepper (1 sliced)
- Green onions (.3 c + 1 T + 1 tsp. chopped)
- Red leaf lettuce (1.6 c)
- Radicchio (1.6 c)
- Escarole (1.6 c)
- Romaine lettuce (3.3 c torn)

What to Do

- In a serving bowl, add in the cherry tomatoes, green pepper, red pepper, red-leaf, scallions, radicchio, escarole and romaine lettuce and combine thoroughly.
- In a separate small bowl whisk in the pepper, salt, lemon juice, vinegar, basil and oil and combine thoroughly.
- Combine the two bowls and toss to and serve.

House Salad

Total Prep & Cooking Time: 15 minutes
Yields: 10 Servings

What to Use

- Pepper (as desired)
- Salt (as desired)
- Parmesan cheese (1 c)
- Red wine vinegar (.5 c)
- Extra virgin olive oil (1 c)
- Pimento peppers (4 oz. diced)
- Red onion (1.6 c)
- Artichoke hearts (14 oz. quartered, drained)
- Iceberg lettuce (1.75 heads torn)
- Romaine lettuce (1.75 heads torn)

What to Do

- ☒ Mix the pimentos, red onions, artichoke hearts and lettuces together and toss to combine.
- ☒ In a small bowl, whisk together the cheese, pepper, salt, red wine vinegar and olive oil. Chill prior to using to top salad. Toss to coat prior to serving.

Chapter 4: Salads for the Entire Family

Sweet potato salad

Total Prep & Cooking Time: 95 minutes
Yields: 4 Servings

What to Use

- Pepper (as desired)
- Salt (as desired)
- Parmigiano-Reggiano cheese (2 in.)
- Baby arugula leaves (.5 lbs.)
- Walnut oil (.5 c)
- Extra virgin olive oil (.5 c)
- Salt (1 tsp.)
- Hot pepper sauce (to taste)
- Dijon mustard (1 tsp.)
- Lemon juice (1 T)
- Shallot (1 chopped)
- Garlic (1 clove minced)
- Red bell peppers (halved)
- Sweet potatoes (4 wedged)
- Olive oil (1 T)

What to Do

- Ensure your oven is heated to 425 degrees F.
- Combine 1 T olive oil with pepper and salt in a small bowl before adding in the sweet potato wedges and tossing to coat.
- Set the bell peppers on a baking sheet and place the sweet potatoes around them.
- Place the baking sheet in the oven for 45 minutes. Shake the pan at the 20 minute mark to prevent sticking.

- ⊠ Add the shallot and garlic to a food processor and process well, add in the pepper, salt, hot sauce, mustard, lemon juice and peppers and process well. Add in the oils and process well.
- ⊠ Add the arugula to a bowl and add in the dressing before tossing well.
- ⊠ Plate the salad, top with potatoes and cheese.

Salad BLT

Total Prep & Cooking Time: 25 minutes
Yields: 6 Servings

What to Use

- Pepper (as desired)
- Salt (as desired)
- Croutons (2 c)
- Tomatoes (2 chopped)
- Romaine lettuce (1 head shredded)
- Garlic powder (1 tsp.)
- Milk (.25 c)
- Mayonnaise (.75 c)
- Bacon (1 lb.)

What to Do

- ⊠ Add the bacon to a skillet before placing the skillet on the stove over a burner turned to a high/medium heat. Let the bacon cook until crisp and then crumble.
- ⊠ In a food processor add together the salt, pepper, garlic powder, milk and mayonnaise and process well.
- ⊠ In a serving bowl, combine the dressing with the croutons, bacon, tomatoes and lettuce and toss to combine prior to serving.

Orzo and spinach salad

Total Prep & Cooking Time: 20 minutes
Yields: 10 Servings

What to Use

- Pepper (as desired)
- Salt (as desired)
- Balsamic vinegar (.5 c)
- Olive oil (.5 c)
- Basil (.5 tsp. dried)
- Pine nuts (.75 c)
- Red onion (.5 chopped fine)
- Feta cheese (.5 lb. crumbled)
- Baby spinach (10 oz. chopped)
- Orzo pasta (16 oz.)

What to Do

- Add the orzo to a pot full of lightly salted water before placing the pot on top of a burner turned to a high heat. Allow the pasta to cook for 8 minutes before draining the pot and running the pasta under cold water.
- In a serving bowl, whisk together the oil, salt, pepper and balsamic vinegar and combine thoroughly.
- Mix in the pasta, pepper, basil, pine nuts, onion and spinach a and toss to combine prior to serving. Top with feta cheese and watermelon and serve.

Asian salad

Total Prep & Cooking Time: 35 minutes
Yields: 6 Servings

What to Use

- Pepper (as desired)
- Salt (as desired)
- Sesame seeds (1 T toasted)
- Green onions (3 chopped)
- Chicken breast (2 halved, shredded, cooked)
- Iceberg lettuce (1 head chopped, dried, rinsed)
- Rice noodles (8 oz. cooked)
- Rice vinegar (3 T)
- Vegetable oil (.25 c)
- Sesame oil (1 T)
- Soy sauce (2 tsp.)
- Brown sugar (2 T)

What to Do

- ☒ In a serving bowl, whisk together rice vinegar, salad oil, sesame oil, soy sauce and brown sugar and combine thoroughly. All the dressing to sit 30 minutes prior to serving.
- ☒ Add the lettuce, sesame seeds, green onions and chicken to the serving bowl and toss well. Allow everything to chill 10 minutes prior to topping with chicken and serving.

Beet salad

Total Prep & Cooking Time: 40 minutes
Yields: 10 Servings

What to Use

- Pepper (as desired)
- Salt (as desired)
- Goat cheese (2 oz.)
- Extra virgin olive oil (.5 c)
- Balsamic vinegar (.25 c)
- Orange juice concentrate (.5 c frozen)
- Mixed greens (10 oz.)
- Maple syrup (3 T)
- Walnuts (.3 c chopped)
- Beets (4 halved)

What to Do

☒ Place the beets in a saucepan and cover them with water before placing them on a burner turned to a high heat. Allow them to cook for 20 minutes before draining the water and cubing them.

☒ Place the walnuts in a skillet and place the skillet on a burner turned to a low/medium heat and allow them to cook until they start to brown before adding in the maple syrup. Coat well and set the walnuts aside.

☒ In a bowl, whisk together the oil, orange juice and balsamic vinegar and combine thoroughly.

☒ Add all of the ingredients, save the goat cheese, to a serving bowl and toss well to combine prior to serving. Plate and top with goat cheese.

Avocado salad with strawberries

Total Prep & Cooking Time: 15 minutes
Yields: 2 Servings

What to Use

- Pepper (as desired)
- Salt (as desired)
- Pecans (.5 c)
- Strawberries (10 sliced)
- Avocado (1 sliced, pitted, peeled)
- Salad greens (2 c torn)
- Lemon juice (1 tsp.)
- Apple cider vinegar (1 T)
- Honey (4 tsp.)
- Olive oil (2 T)
- White sugar (2 T)

What to Do

- ☒ In a serving bowl, whisk together the oil, sugar, honey, lemon juice and vinegar and combine thoroughly.
- ☒ Add the remaining ingredients and toss to coat, chill prior to serving.

Butter lettuce salad with egg

Total Prep & Cooking Time: 55 minutes
Yields: 4 Servings

What to Use

- ☒ Pepper (as desired)
- ☒ Salt (as desired)

- ☒ Chives (.25 c sipped)
- ☒ Butter lettuce (1 head)
- ☒ Lemon juice (2 T)
- ☒ Asparagus (1 lb. chopped)
- ☒ Eggs (4 fried)
- ☒ Sugar (.25 tsp.)
- ☒ Butter (1 stick)
- ☒ Sugar snap peas (8 oz.)
- ☒ Baby potatoes (1 lb.)

What to Do

- ☒ Add the potatoes to a pot and cover them with 2 inches of water before adding a pinch of salt. Place the pot on the stove over a burner turned to a high heat and let it boil before cooking for 10 minutes. Add in the snap peas along with the asparagus and let everything cook about 2 minutes.
- ☒ Drain the pot and slice the potatoes.
- ☒ Add the butter to a saucepan before placing it over a burner turned to a high heat. Whisk in the sugar, lemon juice, salt and pepper.
- ☒ Divide the remaining ingredients between the plates, top with dressing and an egg prior to serving.

Farro salad with cherries

Total Prep & Cooking Time: 30 minutes
Yields: 6 Servings

What to Use

- ☒ Black pepper (as desired)
- ☒ Sea salt (as desired)
- ☒ Parsley (2 T)

- ☒ Dried cherries (.75 c)
- ☒ Green apple (1 c)
- ☒ Basil (.5 tsp dried)
- ☒ Oregano (.5 tsp dried)
- ☒ Farro (1 c)
- ☒ Vegetable broth (2.5 c)
- ☒ Walnuts (.25 c)
- ☒ Salt (.5 tsp)
- ☒ White sugar (2 tsp)
- ☒ Apple cider vinegar (.25 c)
- ☒ Maple syrup (.25 c)
- ☒ Olive oil (.25 c)

What to Do

- ☒ In a small bowl, combine the salt, sugar, vinegar, maple syrup and oil and whisk well.
- ☒ Add the walnuts to a skillet before adding the pan to a burner turned to a low heat for about 3 minutes until they are well toasted.
- ☒ Add the basil, oregano, farro and vegetable broth to a saucepan on top of a burner turned to a high heat. Once it boils, reduce the heat to low/medium and allow everything to simmer about 10 minutes.
- ☒ Remove the saucepan from the burner, and let it sit, covered, for approximately 25 minutes to allow the farro to absorb all of the liquid.
- ☒ Move the farro to a glass bowl and allow it to cool to room temperature before mixing in the walnuts, parsley, dried cherries and green apples. Mix well and place the bowl, covered, into the refrigerator to chill prior to serving.

Chapter 5: Lunch Salads

Classic Mexican Salad

Total Prep & Cooking Time: 75 minutes
Yields: 8 Servings

What to Use

- ☒ Pepper (as desired)
- ☒ Salt (as desired)
- ☒ Hot pepper sauce (as desired)
- ☒ Chili powder (.5 tsp.)
- ☒ Cumin (.5 T ground)
- ☒ Cilantro (.25 c chopped)
- ☒ Garlic (1 clove crushed)
- ☒ White sugar (2 T)
- ☒ Lemon juice (1 T)
- ☒ Lime juice (2 T)
- ☒ Red wine vinegar (.5 c)
- ☒ Olive oil (.5 c)
- ☒ Red onion (1 chopped)
- ☒ Corn kernels (10 oz. frozen)
- ☒ Red bell pepper (1 chopped)
- ☒ Green bell pepper (1 chopped)
- ☒ Cannellini beans (15 oz. rinsed, drained)
- ☒ Kidney beans (15 oz. rinsed, drained)
- ☒ Black beans (15 oz. drained, rinsed)

What to Do

- ☒ In a serving bowl, combine the red onion, frozen corn, bell peppers and beans and mix well.

- ☒ In a smaller separate bowl combine the pepper, cumin, cilantro, hot pepper sauce, garlic, salt, sugar, lemon juice, lime juice, red wine vinegar and olive oil and whisk well.
- ☒ Pour the dressing over the salad and toss well to coat, cover the salad with plastic wrap and allow it to chill in the refrigerator and serve chilled.

Classic Caesar Salad

Total Prep & Cooking Time: 35 minutes
Yields: 6 Servings

What to Use

- ☒ Pepper (as desired)
- ☒ Salt (as desired)
- ☒ Romaine lettuce (1 head torn)
- ☒ Bread (4 cups stale, cubed)
- ☒ Olive oil (.25 c)
- ☒ Lemon juice (1 T)
- ☒ Dijon mustard (1 tsp.)
- ☒ Worcestershire sauce (1 tsp.)
- ☒ Parmesan cheese (6 T grated, divided)
- ☒ Anchovy fillets (5 minced)
- ☒ Mayonnaise (.75 c)
- ☒ Garlic (6 cloves peeled, divided)

What to Do

- ☒ Mince the 3 garlic cloves before adding them to a small bowl along with the lemon juice, mustard, Worcestershire sauce, 2 T parmesan cheese, anchovies and mayonnaise and combining thoroughly. Season as desired before refrigerating the dressing.

- ☒ Add the oil to a skillet before placing it on a burner turned to a medium heat. Cut the rest of the garlic into quarters and add it to the skillet. Allow it to brown before removing it from the pan and adding in the bread instead. Brown the bread and season as desired.
- ☒ Combine all of the ingredients and toss to coat.

Classic black bean salad

Total Prep & Cooking Time: 25 minutes
Yields: 6 Servings

What to Use

- ☒ Pepper (as desired)
- ☒ Salt (as desired)
- ☒ Green onions (6 sliced)
- ☒ Tomatoes (2 chopped)
- ☒ Red bell pepper (1 chopped)
- ☒ Avocado (1 diced, pitted, peeled)
- ☒ Corn kernels (1.5 c)
- ☒ Black beans (30 oz. drained rinsed)
- ☒ Cayenne pepper (as desired)
- ☒ Garlic (1 clove minced)
- ☒ Olive oil (.5 c)
- ☒ Lime juice (.3 c)

What to Do

- ☒ Combine the onions, tomatoes, bell pepper, avocado corn and beans in a serving bowl and mix well.
- ☒ Add the cayenne pepper, salt, pepper, garlic, olive oil and lime juice to a small jar, cover the jar with a lid and shake well.

☒ Toss with dressing as desired.

Buttermilk chicken salad

Total Prep & Cooking Time: 30 minutes
Yields: 4 Servings

What to Use

- Pepper (as desired)
- Salt (as desired)
- Romaine lettuce (2 heads torn)
- Olive oil (1 T)
- Chicken breast (24 oz.)
- Parmesan cheese (.25 c)
- Lemon juice (2 T)
- Radicchio (.5 sliced thin)
- Mayonnaise (.25 c)
- Multigrain bread (2 slices)
- Garlic clove (1 pressed)
- Buttermilk (1.5 c)

What to Do

- Mix together the parmesan cheese, garlic, lemon juice and buttermilk and combine thoroughly before seasoning with salt and pepper as desired.
- Add all of the results, expect for .5 c, to a large Ziploc bag before adding in the chicken and shaking to coat. Allow the chicken to sit for up to 24 hours.
- Place the chicken on a foil-lined baking sheet and broil it for 14 minutes or until it reaches an internal temperature of 165 degrees F.
- Combine all of the ingredients in a serving bowl, top with the remaining buttermilk and toss to combine.

Taco salad

Total Prep & Cooking Time: 30 minutes
Yields: 6 Servings

What to Use

- Pepper (as desired)
- Salt (as desired)
- Cherry tomatoes (1 c halved)
- Boston lettuce (2 heads, leaves separated)
- Green salsa (1.5 c)
- Zucchini (1 diced)
- Onion (1 diced)
- White cheddar cheese (1 c shredded)
- Tortilla chips (1.5 c crushed)
- Red bell pepper (1 diced)
- Turkey (1 lb. ground)
- Olive oil (4 T)

What to Do

- Add 2 T oil to a skillet before placing it on the stove over a burner turned to a high/medium heat. Add in the onion and allow it to cook for about 5 minutes before mixing in the turkey and allowing it to cook about 5 minutes.
- Mix in 1 c salsa, red bell pepper and zucchini and cook another 5 minutes, season as desired and remove the skillet from the stove.
- Combine the remaining ingredients in a serving bowl and mix well before plating. Top with the turkey and then the cheese prior to serving.

Spinach salad and poppy dressing

Total Prep & Cooking Time: 15 minutes
Yields: 10 Servings

What to Use

- Pepper (as desired)
- Salt (as desired)
- Almonds (1.25 c slivered)
- Red onion (.75 c + 1 T + 1 tsp. sliced thin)
- Mandarin oranges (10 oz. drained)
- Salad greens (10 c)
- Baby spinach (10 c)
- Poppy seeds (2.5 tsp.)
- White sugar (.75 c + 1 T + 1 tsp.)
- White vinegar (.75 c + 1 T + 1 tsp.)
- Miracle Whip (1.25 c)

What to Do

- In a serving bowl, whisk together the salt, pepper, vinegar, poppy seeds, sugar and Miracle Whip and combine thoroughly.
- Mix in the almonds, onion, oranges, salad greens and spinach leaves and combine well. Toss to combine prior to serving.

Pomegranate and pear salad

Total Prep & Cooking Time: 12 minutes
Yields: 10 Servings

What to Use

- Pepper (as desired)
- Salt (as desired)
- Honey (2 T)
- Dijon mustard (1.5 T)
- Lemon juice (.25 c)
- Pomegranate juice (1.6 c)
- Vegetable oil (.25 c)
- Pomegranate seeds (1.6 c)
- Anjou pear (5)
- Green leaf lettuce (15 c)

What to Do

- Split the lettuce into 10 bowls, divide the pear slices and the pomegranate seeds between them and mix well.
- Separately whisk together the oil, salt, pepper, honey, mustard, pomegranate juice and lemon juice in a saucepan before placing the pan on a burner turned to a high heat. Once it boils, reduce the heat and allow it to simmer, stir regularly until the sauce thickens. Pour dressing over salad and serve.

Conclusion

Congratulations! And thank for making it through to the end of this book, let's hope it was informative and able to provide you with all of the tools you need to achieve your goals whatever they may be.

** Remember to use your link to claim your 3 FREE Cookbooks on Health, Fitness & Dieting Instantly

https://bit.ly/2MkqTit

Lightning Source UK Ltd.
Milton Keynes UK
UKHW020633200421
382299UK00011B/758

9 781913 540388